I0439388

TABLE OF CONTENTS

Anti Aging Techniques EXPOSED Vol 4
Stopping the Clock with Diet & Nutrition
©Copyright 2013 by Dr. Noah Pranksky

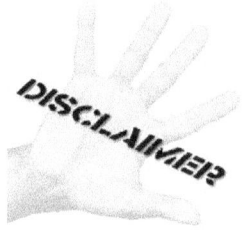

DISCLAIMER AND TERMS OF USE AGREEMENT:

(Please Read This Before Using This Book)

This information is for educational and informational purposes only. The content is not intended to be a substitute for any professional advice, diagnosis, or treatment.

The authors and publisher of this book and the accompanying materials have used their best efforts in preparing this book.

The authors and publisher make no representation or warranties with respect to the accuracy, applicability, fitness, or completeness of the contents of this book. The information contained in this book is strictly for educational purposes. Therefore, if you wish to apply

Introduction – The Retardation of Aging

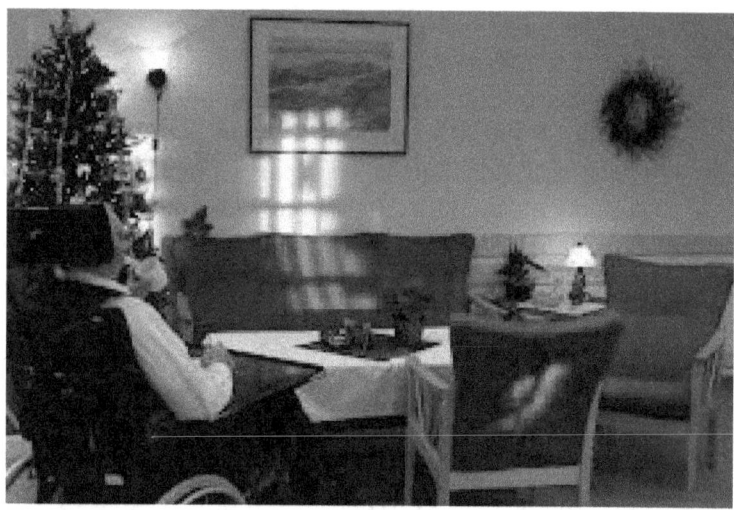

In this volume I want to address the retardation of aging in more detail. In my previous volumes, I demonstrated the science of aging, the mysteries of aging, and the cause of aging and how to use various techniques to increase your energy and vitality that aging takes away.

The science of aging is a dynamic field of study. There is nothing static about it! Every day, social scientists worldwide are locked in constant battle over the various components of the aging equation.

Everything from eternal life and the fountain of youth, to social arguments that aging is mandatory for the human species to survive, are debated and fought over in symposiums, scientific journals, white papers, and more.

But as I describe in one of my previous volumes, aging, beauty, and contentment are a lot more than the realm of the physical. The internal YOU has a good deal to do with it too.

All of the social arguments notwithstanding, the concept of aging is how YOU view it and whatever component of aging is important to YOU!

My personal take on aging leans more toward the quality of life side of the equation rather than the physical or beauty side and as I get older the vanity in me seems to have disappeared as I pay more attention to feeling fit and mentally alert.

But as the saying goes, "To each his own," and whatever part of the aging equation interests you the most, my goal is to be sure you are armed with the proper information to satisfy your interests.

Before I move on, I would like to share with you something I found while rummaging around in my research papers. I think it will cause you to pause and think. It is the opening prologue to a book about a woman who is "going through a middle age crisis" and is fed up with her family and marriage and decides to go seek the wild life. Here it is...

"The Mask"

He walks alone, heartbroken
A union severed, a family lost
Thinking now his life lacks purpose
Isn't this the ultimate cost?

The woman quickly forgets their memories
Helped along by frequent guests
As the man struggles with his own existence
To raise his daughters and forget the past

But time changes all pictures
What was once desirable, is now routine
The woman's memories rise within her
To plague her mind with family scenes

She remembers happiness, remembers sorrow
Looks at pictures stained with tears
The woman tires of constant activity
And longs for faithful love with endless years

So she changes her appearance
Masks her feelings and her soul
And goes out to reacquire
What she had and what she let go

The man is truly smitten
How familiar she does seem
Is it be possible to find another
With the ledger of his sins?

He finds himself still thinking
She is pretty; she is not
As he stares at the mask of beauty

With the drunkenness of a sot

It takes the man awhile
To recognize the fraud in which he sees
He smiles gently at the lady and says,
"My dear, the mask is me!"

In this story, the woman leaves her marriage and family to seek another life but quickly tires of it and in order to get her husband back; she has plastic surgery and changes her physical appearance. Then she goes and attempts to rekindle the relationship. Her husband is truly smitten but quickly discovers her plot. She had attempted to "mask" her appearance and portray something she was not. But when her husband saw through it, he then realized that the goodness that her mask falsely portrayed was his goodness. He was the real person, the loving father and she was just a facade.

In presenting this story to you, I wanted you to see a simple idea here. The retardation of age is important for various reasons to each person that addresses this issue. Please make sure that it is never a mask for something other than what is real. To this author, the beauty of a person resides more inside than outside. I want to look to the heart of a person; everything else is just a facade!

Chapter 1 - Fish Oils and Longevity

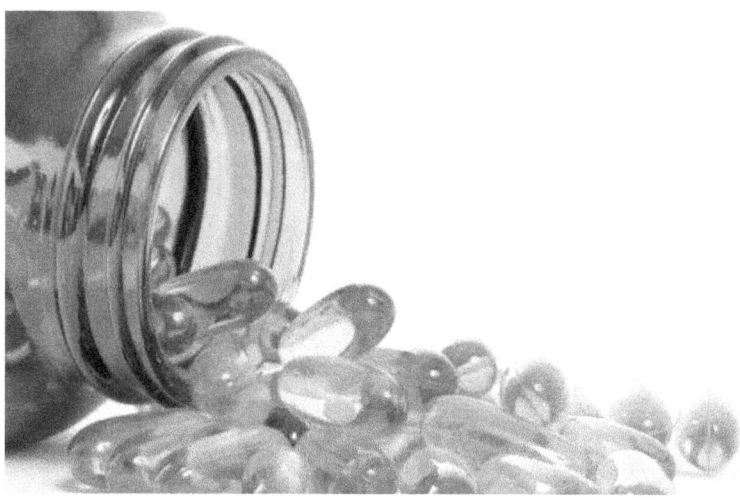

Essential Fatty Acids

When people say the word "FAT" they immediately think of a food that could add unsightly pounds to their waistline, causing them to gain unnecessary weight. This is just plain wrong! There are "good" fats and "bad" fats and the beneficial ones can actually help decrease the desire to eat the harmful ones. Fats do many things for the body.

Fats, also known as "lipids", are the body's prime source of energy (not carbs).

They balance the body's chemistry and help with the transportation and absorption of fat-soluble vitamins such as vitamins A, D, E, and K. But their most important function is as a source of the vital nutrients known as essential fatty acids (EFAs). Essential Fatty Acids are vital to our body's need for many functions. They are found in seeds of plants and in oils of cold-water fish. EFAs are sometimes referred to as Vitamin F. Since our bodies cannot make EFAs, they must be supplied by our diet. Here is a list of the vital functions EFAs accomplish in our bodies:

- Lowers triglyceride levels.
- Helps eradicate plaque from arterial walls.
- Lowers blood pressure.
- Alters the production of leukotrienes, which aggravate inflammation in the body. This is good news to those suffering from arthritis, lupus, psoriasis and other inflammation-related ailments.
- Helps to construct body membranes working with cholesterol and protein to repair old cell membranes and construct new ones.
- Helps to strengthen cell and capillary structures.
- Prolongs blood-clotting time.
- Helps in the manufacture of hemoglobin, the compound in the blood that provides oxygen to the cells from the lungs.
- Assists in the manufacture of cholesterol and also removes excess cholesterol from the blood. Cholesterol has gotten some undeserved press. Cholesterol is a waxy alcohol and is necessary for many vital bodily functions. Interestingly enough, there is no known cholesterol-sensing mechanism in the body. This tells us that an abundance of cholesterol is not a cause for alarm. It is found in the bile, blood, brain tissue, liver, kidneys, adrenal glands, and the myelin sheath of nerve fibers. It

helps absorb and transport EFAs and is necessary for the body to synthesize vitamin D. All hormones are made from cholesterol. The body will actually manufacture cholesterol from dietary by-products of proteins, sugars and fats (by cells, glands, the small intestine and the liver) to insure a continuous supply of this important fat. If your diet contains excessive saturated fats, the body will convert them into cholesterol. People who eat high sugar or fat diets may therefore experience elevated cholesterol levels.

- Prevents the growth of bacteria and viruses, which will not thrive in the presence of oxygen, by oxygenating cell membranes. Highly unsaturated fatty acids have the ability to hold oxygen and this results in increasing resistance to disease, increased endurance, better metabolic efficiency and energy conversion, plus the balancing of sleep-wake cycles. And for you workout nuts, EFAs also shorten the recovery times for tired muscles.

- Assists in the functions of glands and hormones. (Note: EFAs must be present along with vitamins E and B to produce sex and adrenal hormones.)

- Nourishes skin, hair and nails. EFAs help to eliminate eczema, psoriasis, dandruff, and help prevent hair loss.

- Increases the rate the body burns fat.

- Helps maintain the body's temperature.

- Assists in the body's production of electrical currents vital for a regular heartbeat.

- Acts as a precursor to the production of hormone-like substances called prostaglandins. Prostaglandins are found in almost all body cells and act as catalysts for many physiological processes.

They help prevent abnormal blood clotting and nerve inflammation. Prostaglandins also help promote blood circulation by dilating the blood vessels and improve immune system function. The most beneficial type of prostaglandin is called PGE-1, which balances cholesterol and blood pressure levels, and stimulates the body's production of T-lymphocytes, which strengthen the immune capabilities. Each cell keeps tiny amounts of EFAs and produces prostaglandins from them, as they are needed. The name prostaglandins were coined because these substances were originally found in high amounts in the prostate gland. There are 36 different prostaglandins with a wide range of roles in the body.

"Stress, allergies, disease, and a diet high in fried food, increase the body's need for EFAs"

Let's discuss the types of fats.

Saturated Fats

All fats are composed of carbon, hydrogen, and oxygen molecules. The carbon atoms of fatty acids hold together in a chain-like fashion. These carbon atoms can attach hydrogen to them. When each place that can hold a hydrogen atom is filled and there is no room for even one more atom, they are described as "saturated". The longer the chain, the harder the fat will be and hence, the higher its melting point. These types of "long-chain fatty acids" are found in hard fats such as those in red meat, cheese, sour cream, and palm kernel and coconut oils.

11

Unsaturated Fats:

These fats are called unsaturated because there are at least two adjacent carbon atoms on a chain, which are not attached to hydrogen atoms. When at least two pairs of carbon atoms are empty, it is known as a monounsaturated fatty acid. When two or more sets are empty, then it is referred to as a polyunsaturated fatty acid. Fatty acids are either essential or nonessential. They are essential if the body cannot synthesize them and the only way they can be obtained is through the diet. As far back as the 1930s, researchers discovered that a lack of EFAs in our diets caused poor reproduction, lowered immunity, rough and dry skin, and slow growth

There are basically three essential fatty acids:

1. Linolenic Acid (Alpha-Lenolenic Omega-3.)

The most common forms of Omega-3 are eicosapentaenioic acid (EPA), docisahexaenoic acid (DHA), and alpha-linolenic acid, which come from plants and help create EPA and DHA. Omega-3 is usually derived from fish oils.

Note: Fish Oils containing Omega-3 found in coldwater fish are salmon, bluefish, herring, tuna, and mackerel.

2. Linoleic Acid (Omega-6)

12

This is the most vital of the EFAs. The other two, linolenic and arachidonic acids can be converted from linoleic acid. It is plant derived and in its most common form, gamma-linolenic acid (GLA) it is known to provide the following benefits:

- Helps facilitate weight loss in overweight persons (but not in people who do not need to lose weight).
- Reduces platelet aggregation (abnormal blood clotting).
- Helps reduce symptoms of depression and schizophrenia.
- Alleviates premenstrual syndrome symptoms.
- May help alcoholics overcome their addiction.

Note: Plants that contain Omega-6 are Black Currant Seed Oil, Borage Oils, Flaxseed Oil, and Evening Primrose

3. Arachidonic Acid

Is unique in that it is abundant in brain cells as well as other cells. To the cell membrane, this acid is critical but elsewhere it may not be so beneficial.

EFA Deficiency Symptoms

A lack of Linoleic Acid can cause adverse symptoms including:

- Acne
- Changes in personality or behavior
- Gallbladder dysfunction
- Slow wound healing
- Cardiovascular problems
- Prostate inflammation
- Thirst due to excessive perspiration
- Arthritis
- Miscarriage
- Poor Growth
- Kidney problems
- Muscle Tremors
- Skin disorders
- Sterility in males

A lack of Linolenic Acid can cause adverse symptoms including:
- Poor Growth
- Learning disability
- Tingling in the extremities
- Impaired motor coordination
- Poor Vision

The human body requires forty-five (45) known essential nutrients and it requires linolenic acid (Omega-3) more than any other (at least 6-grams/day). Of the forty-five needed nutrients, 20 are minerals, 15 are vitamins, 8 are amino acids and 2 are fatty acids. Altered fatty acids are called Trans-fatty Acids and are extremely bad for the body. Stay away from deep fried foods. Heated fats, especially of the vegetable kind, may turn into cancer-causing agents by causing free-radical damage to the body. The body CANNOT use trans-fatty acids so they simply collect around fatty tissues and the body's organs. Studies show that EFAs may be helpful for many chronic stubborn conditions. The EFAs' ever growing repertoire of valuable applications includes overcoming diseases such as alcoholism, breast cancer, and cardiovascular disease, strengthening the immune system, helping eliminate yeast infection, reducing symptoms of premenstrual syndrome, minimizing inflammation of rheumatoid arthritis, and assisting in the proper management of weight.

Chapter 2 - The Best Anti-Aging Foods

TOP 10 ANTI-AGING FOODS

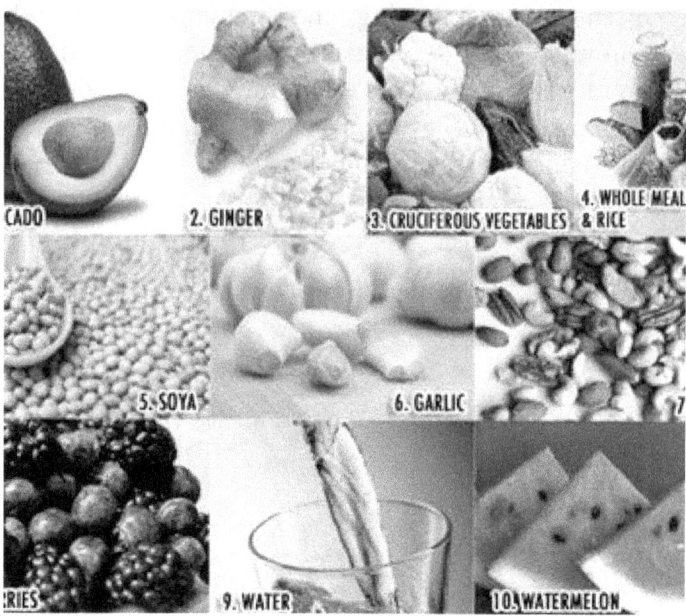

The food and drink options listed below are the best ones that will help your body fight off the damage caused by aging. Use these when you formulate your daily and weekly meal plans and you'll receive extra vitamins, antioxidants and other substances that will help your body fight age-related illnesses and be anti aging resources for you. Start today!

1. Avocados

Avocados lead my list of anti-aging foods because they are just so delicious. Of course, avocados are loaded with healthy fats to help improve your cholesterol, which is the main reason to eat avocados but don't eat too many of them because they are high in calories. The most common and most expensive avocado is called "haas" and you can always recognize it because it has pimply rough skin.

Oddly enough, the most inexpensive and largest avocado ...and also the most flavorful is call "fuerte" and you can recognize it because it is real large and has a smooth skin.

2. Walnuts

I know I need to eat more omega-3s and that fish is a great source, but I have to admit that possible mercury contamination of fish has got me a bit scared off. I deal with this contamination issue in Chapter 4. Walnuts, on the other hand, are a great (and mercury-free) source of omega-3 essential fatty acids. Eat a handful or two a day for all your omega-3 needs.

3. Green Vegetables

President Bush may not like broccoli but it is great stuff! I know vegetables are a touchy subject but we all really need to eat them. In fact, if everyone ate 5 or more servings of fruits and vegetables every day, we'd see a huge decrease in heart disease, cancer, high blood pressure and more. Focus on leafy or deeply colored vegetables for the most benefit.

4. Water

Water is good for you and has been called the fountain of life. There are some nifty arguments in the medical world whether drinking TONS of water is really a good idea, but while they sort that out stay focused on water. Make water your primary drink and be consistent with its intake. You don't need to drink a couple of 8 oz. glasses every hour and tax your kidneys but over the course of a day try to drink at least 6-8 glasses of water.

5. Berries

Berries are full of antioxidants and other chemicals that your body uses to make repairs and prevent damage caused by aging. Best of all, berries taste really, really good. Be sure to eat your berries without any sauces or sugars. Just eat them plain! They are "berry" nice (lol)!

6. Green Tea

Green tea is a longevity supplement in Asia and has been for thousands of years. Green tea contains high concentrations of just the chemicals your body needs. Green tea is also inexpensive, delicious and gives a mild (and gentle) energy boost from its "natural" caffeine.

7. Red Wine

Red wine is good for you -- it contains a substance called "resveratrol" that help your body fight off age-related illnesses. At the end of your day have a glass or two to relax and unwind. You'll get the benefits of a delicious drink along with the anti-aging properties of resveratrol.

8. Beans

Beans are a great source of healthy protein and antioxidants. Some researchers (like T. Colin Powell) believe that animal protein may cause many of the illnesses we face as we age. Switching to a (healthy) more vegetarian diet certainly will help improve the health of your heart and arteries. Beans are a necessary part of any healthy vegetarian diet.

If you don't want to go all the way to vegetarianism, then just start by substituting a few meals a week with bean-based entrees.

9. Melons
Melons have some of the best nutritional profiles of all the fruits. They are pulpy (so they fill you up) and contain lots of vitamins for your body. Work melons into your daily/weekly diet and you'll be reaping health benefits as you enjoy them.

10. Chocolate
Chocolate is good for you but that doesn't mean you should make a meal out of it. It has a balance of fats that don't harm your body and tons of healthy chemicals that your body needs. The only draw-back is that chocolate also has calories. Have a little square every day, but don't overdo it.

Strange Longevity Foods
Anti-aging foods seem to be showing up everywhere with some nutritional claims jumping on the anti aging bandwagon. Learn about noni juice, goji berries, pomegranates and whether they are worth paying extra

for. Here are some nutritional databases and research articles to help you decide.

1. Turmeric - World's Healthiest Spice

Turmeric contains curcumin, a substance under research for multiple health benefits (including cancer prevention/treatment).

You can find turmeric in curries and many Asian dishes. Click on the link below to learn how to gain the health benefits of turmeric — a legitimate superfood.

2. Spirulina - Algae for Health

Spirulina is a name for supplements created from blue-green algae. Spirulina contains all sorts of vitamins and minerals and makes for a good natural supplement to a healthful diet.

Spirulina fans also like to make claims about other health benefits; do they stand up to scrutiny?

3. Noni Juice - Miracle or Scam?

Noni juice has a huge marketing campaign behind it and candidly in my opinion, any food that needs marketing is suspect.

How come you never see many ads for broccoli? The jury is still out on noni juice.

4. Goji Berry - Can Goji Berries Live Up to the Hype?

Goji berries are showing up everywhere along with anti-aging and health claims and it turns out that goji berries live up to some of the hype and don't live up to the rest.

5. Acai Berry - Superfood or Just Another Berry?
Acai berries with all of its health and anti-aging claims have some good and some exaggerated benefits.

6. Pomegranates - Ancient Anti-Aging Secret?
Pomegranates carry an allure of legend and anti-aging properties and they are fairly good for you and can make up part of a healthful, balanced diet.

7. Mushrooms - Fungus for Health
Good old-fashioned mushrooms are a great source of fiber, vitamins, minerals and other nutrients. Add mushrooms in to your diet to help round things out, but be careful to avoid mushrooms grown in chemicals or questionable places.

8. Wheatgrass - The Original Superfood
Wheatgrass may be the original superfood with a history dating back to the early 1900s. You'll find people who grow their own wheatgrass add wheatgrass to smoothies or just take daily shots of juiced wheatgrass. My opinion…good stuff but I didn't come here to graze.

Chapter 3 - The Mediterranean Diet and Living Longer

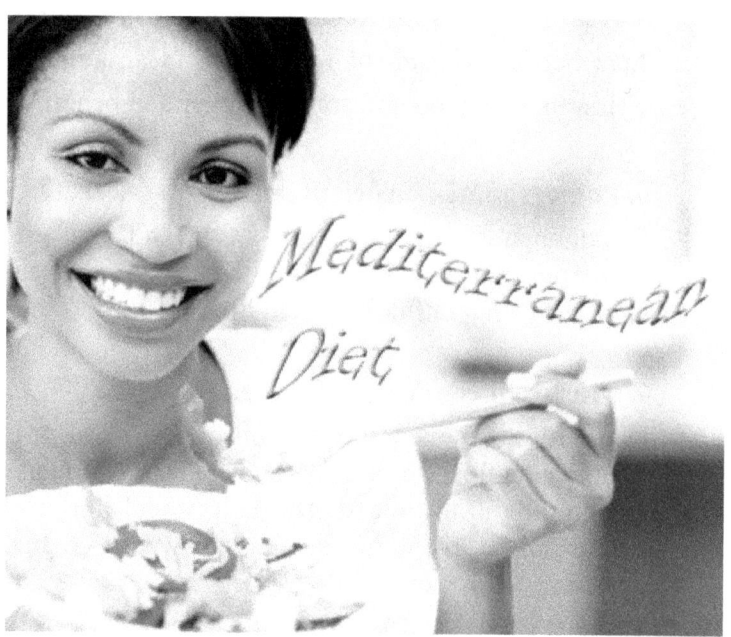

The Mediterranean Diet utilizes the idea that there are certain regions of the world where life expectancy is high and people age well. If we eat what they eat, we'll live longer and age better too. This gave birth to the Mediterranean Diet craze. Now you can find books, cookbooks, websites and more all dedicated to the Mediterranean Diet.

What is the Mediterranean Diet?

It is a diet that consists of vegetables, legumes (beans), fruits, nuts, whole grains, fish, moderate alcohol, a high ratio of monounsaturated fats to saturated fats (lots of olive oil) and lean meat (chicken). Basically, it comes down to lots of vegetables cooked in olive oil, nuts and beans and not very much dairy and meat -- they are more of a side dish.

Does it Increase Life Expectancy?

Yes. In a study of 214,284 men and 166,012 women, researchers were able to look at how closely these people followed the Mediterranean Diet and the impact it had on their life expectancy.

The study took place for ten years (1995 to 2005). Over that time period, 27,799 people in the study died. Researchers were able to use food surveys to classify how closely people followed the Mediterranean Diet.

They found that for both men and women, people who ate closely to the Mediterranean Diet had lower chances of dying from cancer or from all causes. These reductions were around 12 to 20%.

This gives some pretty convincing evidence that following the Mediterranean Diet is a good thing, although it is possible that people who follow any diet are less likely to die because these people are most likely to be careful about their health.

Researchers were able to remove smokers from the analysis (it did not change the results), but you have to wonder if people who are eating close to the Mediterranean Diet are different from other people in more than food choices.

Get Started on the Mediterranean Diet

The real key to the Mediterranean Diet is vegetables, lots and lots of vegetables. Start by adding 2 servings of vegetables to your diet this week. Keep adding them and replacing meat and other foods (such as potato chips) with vegetables. Read more about adding 2 servings and living longer.

One note: The benefits of the Mediterranean diet aren't so great if you don't also have a Mediterranean active lifestyle. Diet is only part of the equation; you must maintain a healthy weight and get regular physical activity too if you want to increase your shot at a long and healthy life.

Let's get back to Chocolate Being Healthy!!!

Why is Dark Chocolate Healthy?

Chocolate is made from plants, which means it contains many of the health benefits of dark vegetables. These benefits are from flavonoids, which act as antioxidants. Antioxidants protect the body from aging caused by free radicals, which can cause damage that leads to heart disease. Dark chocolate contains a large number of antioxidants (nearly 8 times the number found in strawberries). Flavonoids also help relax blood pressure through the production of nitric oxide, and balance certain hormones in the body.

Heart Health Benefits of Dark Chocolate:

Dark chocolate is good for your heart. A small bar of it every day can help keep your heart and cardiovascular system running well. Two heart health benefits of dark chocolate are:

- Lower Blood Pressure: Studies have shown that consuming a small bar of dark chocolate everyday can reduce blood pressure in individuals with high blood pressure.
- Lower Cholesterol: Dark chocolate has also been shown to reduce LDL cholesterol (the bad cholesterol) by up to 10 percent.

Other Benefits of Dark Chocolate:

Chocolate also holds benefits apart from protecting your heart:

- it tastes good
- it stimulates endorphin production, which gives a feeling of pleasure
- it contains serotonin, which acts as an anti-depressant
- it contains theobromine, caffeine and other substances which are stimulants

Doesn't Chocolate Have a lot of Fat?

Here is some more good news -- some of the fats in chocolate do not impact your cholesterol. The fats in chocolate are 1/3 oleic acid, 1/3 stearic acid and 1/3 palmitic acid:

- **Oleic Acid** is a healthy monounsaturated fat that is also found in olive oil.
- **Stearic Acid** is a saturated fat but one which research is shows has a neutral effect on cholesterol.
- **Palmitic Acid** is also a saturated fat, one which raises cholesterol and heart disease risk.

That means only 1/3 of the fat in dark chocolate is bad for you.

Chocolate Tip 1 - Balance the Calories:

This information doesn't mean that you should eat a pound of chocolate a day. Chocolate is still a high-calorie, high-fat food. Most of the studies done used no more than 100 grams, or about 3.5 ounces, of dark chocolate a day to get the benefits. One bar of dark chocolate has around 400 calories. If you eat half a bar of chocolate a day, you must balance those 200 calories by eating less of something else. Cut out other sweets or snacks and replace them with chocolate to keep your total calories the same.

Chocolate Tip 2 - Taste the Chocolate:

Chocolate is a complex food with over 300 compounds and chemicals in each bite. To really enjoy and appreciate chocolate, take the time to taste it. Professional chocolate tasters have developed a system for tasting chocolate that include assessing the appearance, smell, feel and taste of each piece.

Chocolate Tip 3 - Go for Dark Chocolate:

Dark chocolate has far more antioxidants than milk or white chocolate. These other two chocolates cannot make any health claims. Dark chocolate has 65 percent or higher cocoa content.

Chocolate Tip 4 - Skip the Nougat:

You should look for pure dark chocolate or dark chocolate with nuts, orange peel or other flavorings. Avoid anything with caramel, nougat or other fillings. These fillings are just adding sugar and fat which erase many of the benefits you get from eating the chocolate.

Chocolate Tip 5 - Avoid Milk:

It may taste good but some research shows that washing your chocolate down with a glass of milk could prevent the antioxidants being absorbed or used by your body.

Chapter 4 - Best Fish for Health

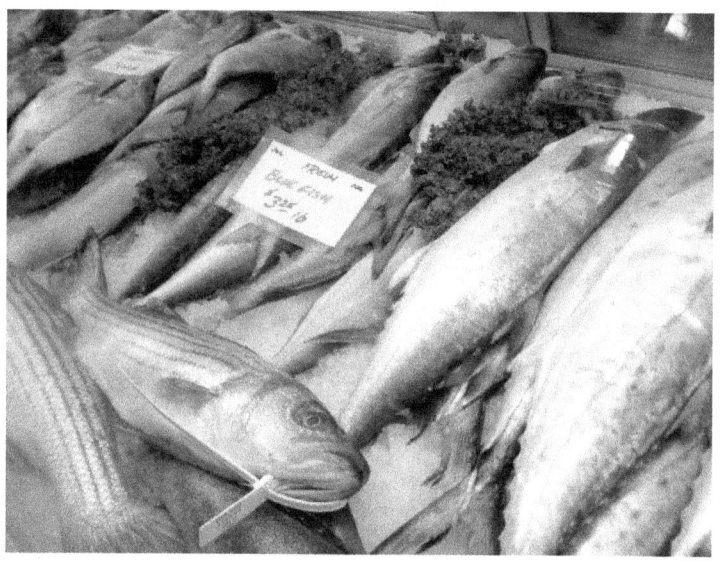

We know that eating fish is good for you. In fact, fish may be the ultimate anti-aging superfood, but eating the wrong kinds of fish too often can raise the level of mercury in your body.

This is especially dangerous for pregnant and breastfeeding women because fetuses and newborns are very sensitive to mercury. Find out the best fish to eat and in what amounts.

Why Eat Fish?

Fish are a great source of protein. They contain healthy fats that will reduce your cholesterol and improve your health. Fish also contain omega-3 fatty acids that help keep your heart healthy and may even improve your mood. Fish have been shown to be an important diet of many long-lived peoples around the world.

The Problem With Fish

All fish contain trace amounts of mercury. For most people, the small amounts in fish do not pose a health problem. Some fish, however, contain high amounts of mercury -- enough to damage a fetus or newborn. That is why pregnant and nursing mothers must be very careful about the amounts and types of fish they eat. Young children should also avoid eating fish high in mercury. According to the FDA, pregnant women and small children (under 6) should not eat more than 2 servings of fish each week -- and should only eat those fish with low mercury content (see below). Mercury levels can build in adults too -- eventually becoming harmful to health. High mercury levels can cause permanent damage to the kidneys and brain.

Which Fish Have the Most Mercury?

Big fish have more mercury for the simple reason that big fish usually live longer. They have more time to build up higher levels of mercury in their bodies. The Environmental Protection Agency (EPA) recommends checking local advisories for the mercury content of fish caught in your area using this website. See the lists below for general mercury levels of many common types of fish and how much of each type to eat (according to the National Resource Defense Council):

LOWEST MERCURY

Eat 2-3 servings a week (pregnant women and small children should not eat more than 12 ounces (2 servings):

- Anchovies
- Catfish
- Clam
- Crab
- Crawfish
- Flounder
- Haddock
- Herring
- Mackerel
- Mullet
- Oyster
- Perch
- Pollock
- Salmon
- Sardine
- Scallop
- Shrimp
- Sole
- Squid
- Tilapia
- Trout
- Whitefish

MODERATE MERCURY

Eat six servings or fewer per month (pregnant women and small children should avoid these):

- Bass
- Carp

- Cod
- Halibut
- Lobster
- Mahi Mahi
- Monkfish
- Perch
- Snapper
- Tuna (Canned Chunk light)

HIGH MERCURY

Eat three servings or less per month (pregnant women and small children should avoid these):

- Bluefish
- Grouper
- Sea Bass
- Tuna (Canned Albacore, Yellowfin)

HIGHEST MERCURY

Avoid eating (everyone):

- Marlin
- Orange Roughy
- Shark
- Swordfish
- Tilefish
- Tuna (Ahi)

Calorie Restriction - Eat Less, Live Longer

Calorie Restriction:

Calorie restriction is a strategy to increase life expectancy by reducing the total amount of calories consumed daily.

31

Calorie restriction research has been around since the 1930s and recent studies have shown longevity benefits to rats and other animals from a low calorie diet.

Calorie restriction is thought to prevent or improve numerous health conditions, especially ones related to cardiovascular disease and diabetes.

Quality, Low Calorie Foods:

In calorie restriction, nutritional choices are very important. Calorie-poor, nutrient-dense foods such as vegetables are chosen over sugars, high carbohydrate items and other foods. Anyone using a calorie restriction diet should be well-educated on nutrition and have regular check-ups with their doctor.

On average, the typical American consumes between 2000 and 3000 calories per day. Someone practicing calorie restriction may consume between 1500 and 2000 daily calories.

Animal Experiments:

The maximum lifespan of rats has been nearly doubled in some experiments by placing the rats on a nutritious, low calorie diet. Other animals have also been used to prove the benefits of calorie restriction including monkeys, mice, and spiders. Not only do the animals on calorie restriction live longer, they remain more youthful, energetic and healthy.

Human Effectiveness:

In humans, calorie restriction has been shown to lower blood pressure, improve the function of heart, veins, and arteries, and lower blood insulin levels. No one really knows if calorie restriction can increase the life expectancy in humans.

Chapter 5 - Red Wine's Anti-Aging Benefits

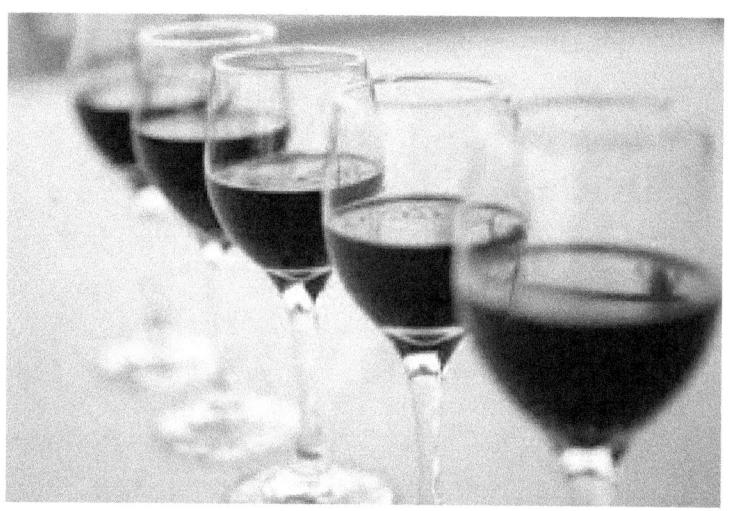

Red wine has been getting a lot of good press for its anti-aging properties. Studies in rats have shown that resveretrol, a substance found in red wine, has strong anti-aging effects. Researchers are beginning to understand why red wine seems to slow aging, especially the aging of the heart.

Why Red Wine Could Keep You Young

In the body, red wine seems to work in a way similar to calorie restriction. When primates and rodents are given a diet which is at 30% less in daily calories, they live longer and are resistant to many age-related problems (calorie restriction is not yet proven in humans).

Not only do the calorie restricted animals live longer, the life span of the animals (the actual span for the species) is increased by 30%. In other words, the oldest monkeys and rats never had a calorie restricted diet. The anti-aging properties of red wine may work through the same mechanism as calorie restriction.

Mice and Red Wine

Middle-aged mice were given low doses of resveratrol (lower than in prior studies) and still showed solid anti aging benefits. What happens is that both calorie restriction and resveratrol supplementation change the activity of certain genes in your body.

These changes result in less age-related problems and a reduction in tissue changes due to aging. The effect was greatest in slowing heart aging. Specifically, situins (a type of enzyme works to make these favorable changes in genes) seems to be stimulated by resveratrol.

How Much Red Wine Should I Drink?

The current laboratory dose of research used in most studies to extend the life of lab rats is the equivalent of 100 bottles of red wine a day for humans. Some studies show that just 30 bottles of wine a day may have benefits. That still is far too high to be of practical use so researchers are hard at work to create a drug to simulate the effects of resveratrol.

Can Supplements Help You Live Longer?

The idea that you can take something to extend your life is seductive, especially given the vast array of vitamins and mineral supplements on the market. Seems simple:

more nutrients = more years. At a time when we're all being told we should eat more fruits and vegetables, are supplements a hedge against a diet that's lacking? Because there are nutrients that you require as you get older to keep your body healthy and disease-free, many people turn to the supplement industry -- with sales hitting 23.7 billion dollars in 2007. Despite this, research continues to be divided on whether individual supplements improve longevity, are harmful, or simply excreted right out of your body. So what should you do, for a longer, healthy life? First of all, remember that the best source of any ingredient is food. Diets rich in beta-carotene have been associated with a lower risk of cancer, for example, but the same protective effect was not found with beta-carotene supplements. Here are some supplements commonly taken for longevity, and the research associated with them:

Calcium: This mineral keeps bones strong and is necessary for muscle and nerve function and blood transport. In a 2011 review of the Iowa Women's Health Study, in which 38,000 older women were tracked over a 22-year period, calcium was the only common multivitamin component shown to have a positive effect on mortality -- that is, those women taking calcium (average 400-1300 mg/day) had a slightly lower risk of dying during that time. By contrast, other reviews of longitudinal or long-term studies have suggested that taking calcium supplements can increase the risk of heart attack and stroke in women. In light of conflicting research, it's best to talk to your doctor about the safety of calcium supplements.

Vitamin D: Vitamin D works with calcium to keep bones healthy; it may also help protect against certain cancers and other diseases. It's synthesized in skin in the presence of UV light, so concerns have been raised about whether people living in northern climates with reduced daylight in winter can get enough. A 2007 review of more than 57,000 participants, in 18 separate research trials, concluded that a safe level of Vitamin D supplementation (400 – 600 IU) did enhance longevity, either by reducing the incidence of certain cancers and cardiovascular disease, or by improving survival in patients with these conditions.

Vitamin B6: Vitamin B is involved in the creation of neurotransmitters and blood cells, and regulating levels of an amino acid called homocysteine. Because B vitamins like folic acid, B6, and B12 have been shown to lower homocysteine levels -- a status associated with a lesser risk of heart disease and stroke -- researchers have investigated whether supplementation would help prevent these conditions and improve longevity. In several large-scale studies, however, these B vitamins as supplements had no effect on the incidence, or severity, of heart disease or stroke. Similarly, in research examining the effect of B6 supplements on the incidence of cancer, no effect on mortality was found.

Vitamin B12: People over the age of 50 may not absorb vitamin B12 -- required for blood and nerve health -- as effectively. Previously, it was believed that vitamin B12 (like B6) supplementation, especially when combined with folic acid, could help ward off heart disease and stroke, but that has largely been discounted. Research is ongoing to see if vitamin B12 can help treat or prevent dementia, which could in turn promote longevity.

Vitamin C: Necessary for the manufacture of collagen and certain neurotransmitters, Vitamin C is also a powerful antioxidant. A 2009 study of more than 77,000 people, between the ages of 50 and 76 years, found that non-smokers who took about 300mg of vitamin C for 10 years were 24% less likely to die during that time period; however, no longevity benefit from taking vitamin C was found for smokers in this group. Research is ongoing to determine whether vitamin C will help prevent certain cancers and cardiovascular disease.

Selenium: A trace mineral, selenium is used to form antioxidant enzymes in the body. Antioxidants mop up the harmful byproducts of cell metabolism and environmental toxin exposure. Selenium levels in populations vary according to the concentration of the mineral in soil where food is grown. A 2008 review of almost 14,000 participants in the United States found a non-linear relationship between levels of selenium in the blood and mortality -- that is, low levels of selenium were associated with higher mortality, as were high levels. Most studies have considered supplements in the range of 100-200mcg; federal dietary guidelines suggest that adults over the age of 19 should consume daily totals of 55 mcg/day, not to exceed 400 mcg/day.

Beta-carotene: A form of vitamin A found in colorful fruits and vegetables, diets rich in beta-carotene have been associated with a lower risk of cancer. Studies into beta-carotene supplements have not shown the same results; some have actually indicated an increase in mortality. There is no recommended daily allowance (RDA) for beta-carotene.

Conclusion

Supplement research faces challenges in terms of sorting out other lifestyle factors (or "confounding" aspects) like smoking, likelihood of getting screened for diseases, diet, and exercise. It will probably be some time before science tells us with certainty which vitamins and minerals can help extend our lives, and by how much. Don't despair -- remember that many studies have shown that a plant-based Mediterranean-style diet delivers on the necessary nutrients for most people. Make sure you consult your physician or nutritionist before taking any supplements. More is not better, so don't mega dose. Vitamins and minerals from all sources (fortified foods, multi-vitamins, single-vitamin products) add up. They can also interfere with medication you may be taking and can be dangerous for people with certain medical conditions.

Resveratrol Supplements - a Fountain of Youth?

Resveratrol supplements seem to be everywhere these days. I see online ads and famous people all talking about them as the "longevity pill" and the "fountain of youth." Dr. Mehmet Oz, Oprah Winfrey and even Barbara Walters are out there talking about resveratrol supplements. What is the truth behind them? Are they worth it?

Resveratrol Supplements

Resveratrol is a substance found in red wine. In extremely high concentrations (the equivalent of 1000 bottles of red wine a day), resveratrol has been shown to combat age-related illness in mice and other animals in the laboratory. Now, everyone seems to be selling a resveratrol supplement and attempting to "cash in" on this new development in anti-aging science.

Resveratrol Supplements - The Truth

The simple truth behind resveratrol supplements is that there is no evidence that these work in humans. Studies are underway, and many very smart people believe that there is something in resveratrol that can help prevent some of the diseases of aging and possibly even extend life. But whether the resveratrol supplements on the market right now are the correct formulations is anyone's guess.

Resveratrol - a $720 Secret

I think of it this way: A few years back, pharma giant GlaxoSmithKline (GSK) bought a company called Sirtris for $720 million dollars. This is the company founded by Dr. Sinclair, one of the leading researchers on resveratrol. I think Glaxo is probably pretty good at determining the worth of a new line of research. I don't think they would have bought Sirtris if all the research was really just about putting high, high concentrations of resveratrol in a supplement. Anyone can do that -- all you have to do is extract enough of it from grapes and other naturally occurring sources (or create it in a lab).

GSK did not pay $720 million for that, they bought something else -- something they believe will revolutionize the treatment of age-related illnesses like diabetes. They are spending even more money developing those treatments because they believe they will be able to create a blockbuster drug. Now, I don't think they would have done this if a simple supplement would do the same thing. In other words, I'm skeptical that resveratrol supplements can do everything they claim. All the websites on the resveratrol supplements point to studies that used different formulations and substances and then make a claim about the product that is being sold.

Resveratrol - Should I Take Some?

That is a harder question. There are some known problems with resveratrol. As with anything you put in your body in such high concentrations, there are likely to be interactions and problems depending on your situation.

There is not a lot known right now about any side effects or drug interactions with resveratrol, but it would be a miracle if there were none. There are some indications that women with estrogen-sensitive cancers should avoid resveratrol, as well as some thinking that resveratrol can interfere with medications like calcium channel antagonists.

There is also the issue of cost -- these pills cost $2 to $4 per daily dose. But on the flip side, they promise healthy aging. So this is a tough decision. You are going to have to research each of your medical conditions and medications, and speak to your doctor, to determine if there might be problem. Then, of course, there is deciding if it's worth your money. Personally, I'll wait until more research comes out.

Chapter 6 - HGH and Aging

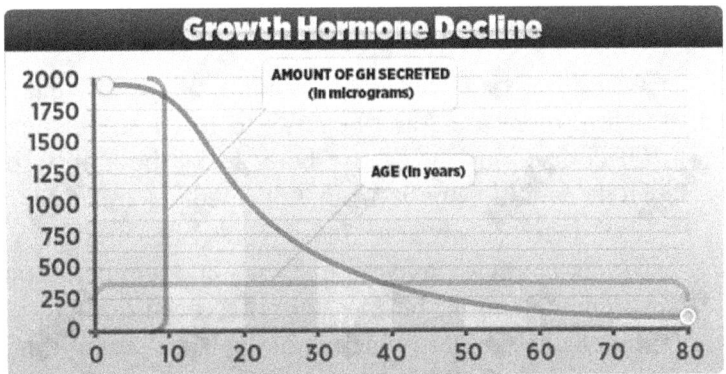

The human growth hormone (HGH) is a hormone that is made by your body in the pituitary gland and many claim has anti aging properties. It is often marketed as an anti-aging hormone. In children, it is important for normal growth. In adults, HGH helps regulate and maintain your tissues and organs. Children sometime receive HGH injections because a lack of HGH in their body is impacting their growth rate.

HGH and Aging

Like many hormones, HGH levels decrease as a person gets older. This is a normal part of aging. HGH is becoming a popular anti-aging supplement. Because HGH is only available in injection form (other forms of HGH have not been proven effective) HGH must be given by a doctor. The cost for one year of HGH injections can be more than $15,000. The saddest part is that there has been little research on HGH and aging --

one study shows that *lower* HGH levels correlate to increased longevity compared to people with high HGH levels.

HGH Benefits

While HGH is not the fountain of youth that people claim, there are some benefits to HGH supplementation. Of course, anyone whose body lacks the ability to make HGH would benefit from this medical treatment. HGH also increase muscle mass (but not strength). Some people claim to have more energy and feel better on HGH supplementation, but no study has been done to rule out the placebo effect (which is likely to be strong if a person is paying $15,000 for treatments).

Why All the Buzz Around HGH?

In 1990, an article appeared in the New England Journal of Medicine by Rudman that showed HGH improved the muscle tone and body composition of 12 older men. That tiny piece of research led to an unexpected boom in quacks and "anti-aging" doctors selling HGH-based "Cures for Aging." Today, there are oral formulas of HGH, injections and even inhaled versions of human growth hormone. Other studies since 1990 have given mixed results. The only firm conclusion is that going to the gym can provide more benefits than HGH (if there are any benefits of HGH at all) with far less cost and risk.

Side Effects of Human Growth Hormone

The side effects of HGH are serious. They include diabetes, swelling, high blood pressure and even heart failure. Inflammation can also occur, causing joint pain and carpel tunnel syndrome. There is also an increased risk of cancer in children using HGH supplementation and a possible increase risk of cancer in adults (though no long-term studies have been done to prove or disprove the cancer risk of HGH).

Conclusion

At the moment, there is not enough evidence to recommend HGH as an anti-aging supplement. This risks, dangers and costs are far too great for anyone to be experimenting with HGH. If you talk with a doctor who recommends HGH for anti-aging, find another doctor (of course, HGH has other valid medical indications like pituitary problems in children).

DHEA for Youth?

DHEA (dehyrdoepiandrosterone) is a hormone made by the body that has become popular for anti aging purposes. DHEA is a raw ingredient that the body can convert into the sex hormones estrogen and testosterone. As a person ages, his or her DHEA level naturally drops. DHEA advocates claim that taking the supplement will slow aging by increasing muscles mass, increasing bone mass, burning fat, amongst other things.

The Evidence – DHEA Supplements Do NOT Slow Aging

A study conducted by the Mayo Clinic, and published in the *New England Journal of Medicine*, showed that DHEA supplementation had no benefit on muscle strength, endurance, glucose tolerance, bone mass, or quality of life.

The study followed 87 men and 57 women over the age of 60 for two years. All of the study participants had low levels of DHEA in their blood before the study began. When participants took supplements of DHEA, the levels of DHEA rose to normal levels. However, this did not translate into any improvements in muscle mass or other measurements.

Scientifically Backed Uses of DHEA Supplements

Fair evidence--DHEA supplements have been shown to benefit some specific conditions, such as adrenal insuffiency and depression. There is also some evidence that DHEA supplementation may assist with weight loss and lupus.

Unclear Evidence--The evidence for using DHEA for the following conditions is not clear, or is contradictory: Alzheimer's disease, bone density, cardiovascular disease, cervical cancer, chronic fatigue syndrome, cocaine withdrawal, Crohn's disease, HIV/AIDS, infertility, menopause, myotonic dystrophy, psoriasis, arthritis, schizophrenia, septicaemia, erectile dysfunction and sexual problems, Sjogren's syndrome, and skin aging.

Evidence Against--Research shows that DHEA used for postmenopausal fibromyalgia, immune stimulation, memory, and muscle strength is either ineffective or counter indicated.

Long-Term Effects

While the *New England Journal of Medicine* study did not show any adverse effects over the two-year period, the sample was very small. No formal studies have been done on the long-term effects of DHEA supplementation. Because it increases the levels of the sex hormones in the body, DHEA supplementation can, in theory, increase the risk of hormone-specific cancers like breast and prostate cancers.

Conclusion

DHEA is not the miracle anti aging supplement that many say it is. There are very specific circumstances in which DHEA can be helpful, but the current evidence does not show any benefit in anti aging.

Anti-Aging Potential of Melatonin 14

Melatonin is a hormone produced in the body that some have claimed to have anti aging properties. It helps regulate your sleep cycle.

When you are exposed to light in the morning, melatonin levels decrease. At night, when it is dark, these levels increase, making you sleepy and drowsy. Some people are claiming that melatonin is an anti-aging hormone.

Melatonin and Aging

There are claims that melatonin levels decrease as we age. These claims are based on the observation that older people need less sleep.

That observation is a common sleep myth. In fact, older people need just as much sleep as younger adults. Melatonin levels, in healthy individuals, do not decrease with age.

Should I Use It to Fall Asleep
Before even thinking about using a supplement to fall asleep, spend about a week re-training your body's sleep habits.

Bad habits like reading in bed, drinking too much caffeine and not getting enough light exposure can result in sleep difficulty.

Re-learn how to fall asleep. If those tips don't work, then you may have a medical condition or may be taking a medication that interferes with sleep. You may also have a sleep disorder. Talk to your doctor about the possibility of changing your medication or treating your sleep problem.

Dosage Warning and Side Effects
Small amounts of melatonin (0.1 to 0.5 milligrams) have been shown to improve sleep in some individuals. Melatonin that is sold over the counter may have doses as high as 3 milligrams. Those doses cause melatonin levels to spike in the body. There is no research on the long-term effects of high levels of melatonin.

Side effects of melatonin can include nightmares, disruption of normal sleep cycles (if taken at the wrong times), headache, daytime drowsiness, gynecomastia (breast enlargement in men), and depression. People who have a history of depression, in particular, should discuss the use of melatonin with their doctors before taking it.

What Can Melatonin Be Used For?

Jet Lag: Studies have shown the melatonin can help reset your body's clock after jet lag. About 50 percent of people in studies were able to reset their body's internal clock faster using low-dose melatonin supplements for a few days.

Delayed Sleep Phase Syndrome: This is a condition in which a person sleeps a normal amount, but their sleep is delayed into late in the night (not because of TV or other reason). Research shows melatonin is promising for treating this syndrome.

Insomnia in the Elderly: Research is also promising (but not proven) that melatonin supplementation can help treat insomnia in older adults. Studies show trends that look good, but the studies were not well-designed and left many questions unanswered. Most studies only looked at short-term effects (a few days).

Sleep Problems in Children with Neuro-Psychiatric Disorders: There is also some promising research that melatonin could help children with conditions such as autism, psychiatric disorders or epilepsy improves their sleep. This use of melatonin is currently being investigated.

Sleep Improvement for Healthy People: There is also good evidence that melatonin helps improve sleep in healthy people. The studies shown that melatonin, taken by mouth about 30 to 60 minutes before sleep, will shorten the time it takes to fall asleep. More research is needed to determine the long-term effects of melatonin supplementation.

Other Uses (unclear evidence):

o improve sleep in people with Alzheimer's disease
o used as an antioxidant
o used to treat ADHD (attention deficit hyperactivity disorder) and ADHD-related sleep problems
o help to taper (stop using) benzodiapepines
o for bipolar disorder-related sleep problems
o in treating cancer (not enough research to know about interference with other treatments and overall effect)
o treatment of chemotherapy side effects
o regulate circadian rhythms in blind persons
o for depression-related sleep disturbances
o to treat glaucoma
o to prevent headaches

Conclusion

There is an increasing interest in using melatonin in many conditions. However, little is known about how high melatonin levels might interact with other therapies. For now, caution should be used. Be sure to talk with your doctor before using melatonin (or any supplement), especially if you have an existing health condition.

Chapter 7 - Selenium to Reduce Cancer Risk

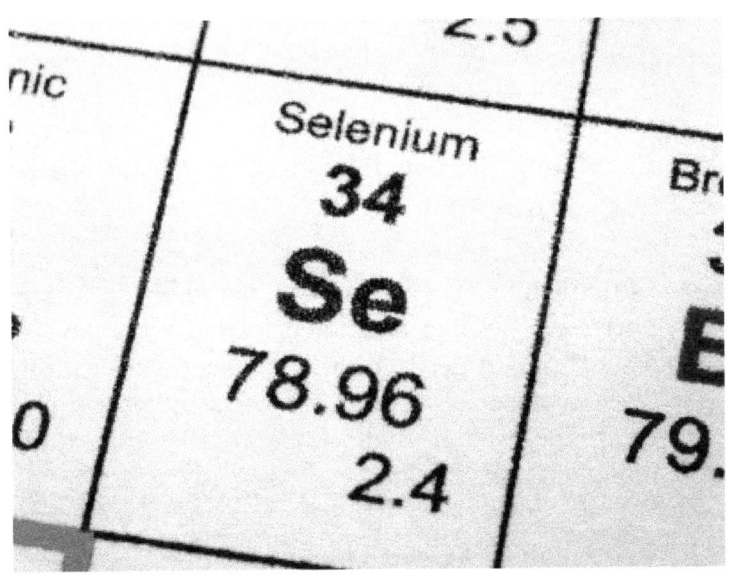

Update: new research puts some doubt on the benefits of selenium and lung cancer prevention. A ten year study led by researchers at the MD Anderson Cancer Center showed no benefit in the prevention of lung cancer. Does that mean selenium is worthless? No -- it just means that it does not look helpful for lung cancer and more research will need to be done to determine other questions (new study source: presentation at the American Society of Clinical Oncology 2010 Annual Meeting by Daniel D. Karp, M.D). You may have heard of selenium as a longevity supplement. It is often promoted as a reducer of cancer and heart disease risk. It works by lessening the negative impact of free radicals in your body. Studies have shown that selenium levels are linked to a reduced risk of prostate and other cancers.

However, there has been some contradictory information that extremely high levels of selenium may actually increase cancer risk.

Examining the Selenium, Cancer, Heart Disease and Longevity Link

To sort this out, researchers conducted a study of almost 14,000 adults. The study examined them selenium levels over 12 years and attempted to link those levels to the overall risk of death, death by cancer and death by heart disease. One of the things the study was trying to determine was if high levels of selenium lead to an increased risk of death.

Too Much of a Good Thing

Researchers found that higher (but not too high) levels of selenium were associated with a decrease in overall death rate and the death rate from cancer. They did not find a link between selenium level and heart disease. Researchers also found that individuals with selenium levels in the blood over 130 ng/ml were more likely to die of cancer. They conclude that moderate increases in selenium level can be linked to increased longevity through a decrease in the risk of cancer and overall death. However, extremely high levels of selenium are no longer helpful and may actually decrease longevity.

Selenium is found in seafood, grains, nuts and other dietary sources. Learn more about selenium as a supplement, its risks and side effects.

Vitamin D Deficiency and Aging

Vitamin D deficiency has been linked to a host of age-related health conditions such as high blood pressure, osteoporosis and even overall mortality. Vitamin D is fast on its way to becoming the "number one vitamin."

Is Vitamin D Really A Vitamin?

Technically, no. Vitamins are micronutrients that the body uses in various processes. Vitamin D is a prohormone, a substance that the body converts into a hormone. But that's a technicality. The thing you need to remember about vitamin D is that your body can make it from sunlight.

Making Vitamin D

What happens is that sunlight (specifically UV-B radiation) hits your skin it reacts with some chemicals (7-dehydrocholesterol) to start making vitamin D. The process is complex and not very interesting. What you need to remember is that around 15 minutes of exposure to sunlight on your hands and face every day is plenty for your body to make enough vitamin D under normal circumstances. If you live up north (or way down south), the atmosphere filters out a lot of the UV-B during winter and you may need more exposure.

What Good Is Vitamin D?

Lots of good, we just don't really know exactly how it works. Vitamin D seems to keep your blood pressure low, reduce inflammation and give the immune system a boost -- all beneficial for keeping your heart health and (maybe) even fighting off cancer. We do know that vitamin D is essential for good bone health -- it helps your bones absorb calcium (and calcium is what bones are made of). Kids without exposure to vitamin D can develop rickets (a disease where their legs become extremely bow-legged) and older adults with vitamin D deficiencies may develop bone diseases.

Research on vitamin D deficiency and depression, vitamin D deficiency and back pain and vitamin D deficiency and heart attacks all show that vitamin D has a larger role to play than just bone health. Vitamin D has been implicated in auto-immune disease too. Diseases like multiple sclerosis may be caused by vitamin D deficiency (according to some theories -- read more on Multiple Sclerosis and Vitamin D).

Types of Vitamin D
Two major forms of vitamin D are vitamin D2 and vitamin D3. Vitamin D2 is also called ergocalciferol and vitamin D3's other name is cholecalciferol. When you look at supplements, most seem to focus on vitamin D3 (cholecalciferol) and you'll see that listed as the ingredient. Read below for more on vitamin D supplementation.

Who is Vitamin D Deficient?
Vitamin D deficiency seems to be common in the U.S. Maybe we are all just spending too much time inside. It is

estimated the 25% of U.S. adults have less than 18 nanograms per milliliter of vitamin D (severe vitamin D deficiency). Overall, 40% of men and 50% of women are thought to be lower than the healthy level of vitamin D (28 nanograms per milliliter). The people most at risk are anyone who spends a lot of time indoors (the elderly and the homebound, for example) and people with dark skin (dark skin absorbs less sunlight).

Vitamin D Deficiency – What Happens in Your Body

When vitamin D levels are low, your body just doesn't seem to work as well. Vitamin D deficiency has been linked to high blood pressure, insulin problems, diabetes risk, obesity and more. Receptors for vitamin D have been found on pancreatic cells that make insulin (leading to a theoretical connection between vitamin D and diabetes). We know that more heart attacks happen in the winter (when people go outside less and therefore have lower vitamin D levels) and that people survive cancer better in the summer (when their vitamin D levels are higher). But we don't fully understand why these things are happening or what exactly vitamin D is doing in the body.

Vitamin D Deficiency and Risk of Death

In a study, records from 13,331 adults from a national survey database compiled by the U.S. government were examined to determine a link between death and vitamin D deficiency (defined as lower than 25-hydroxyvitamin D (25(OH) D). Vitamin D levels were tested from 1988 to 1994 and the people were followed until 2000 for information about cause of death.

On average, people in the study were followed for 8.7 years.

Researchers found that vitamin D deficiency was linked to all-cause mortality. People in with the lowest levels (bottom 25%) of vitamin D had a 26% increase in risk of death during the study period compared to people with the highest levels of vitamin D. This accounted for 3.1% of the mortality risk of the total population.

Because the sample was representative of the total U.S. population, we can generalize from this study to say that 3.1% of deaths in the U.S. are linked to vitamin D deficiency. Researchers believe that vitamin D deficiency is an independent risk factor for heart disease and should be consider with other risk factors like family history, high blood pressure or being overweight. Vitamin D deficiency may also be a factor in cancer deaths as well.

Vitamin D Deficiency and Aging
We know that many older adults have vitamin D deficiencies. The real question is whether the deficiency has something to do with the aging body (for example, the body can't produce sufficient levels of vitamin D anymore) or whether older people's behavior is different (for example, they don't get exposed to much sunlight). This is an important question because it will answer the question of "what do we do about vitamin D deficiency in older adults?"
Researchers Robert Scragg and Carlos Camargo took that same database compiled by the U.S. government used in the study above (the Third NHANES) and looked for a link between vitamin D levels and outdoor activity in

adults. They found that, indeed, vitamin D levels decreased with age.

They also found that participating in outdoor physical activity decreased with age. People aged 60 or more, however that did some daily outdoor activity had the vitamin D levels of a young adult. So the conclusion is that vitamin D levels in the body don't decrease with age, but people's amount of time outdoors does. This is good news. You can keep your vitamin D levels up simply by spending a bit of time outdoors every day.

Vitamin D Deficiency and Arthritis

There even might be a link between vitamin D deficiency and rheumatic diseases like arthritis. A doctor at a rheumatology clinic has all new patients tested for vitamin D deficiency. After testing 231 patients, he found that 162 (70%) had low levels of vitamin D and 26% had severe vitamin D deficiency. Unfortunately, this is just an observation. We don't know what the average for that town is or is rheumatic diseases may impact vitamin D levels (for example, people with rheumatic diseases may stay indoors more because they don't feel good). It was also not mentioned if giving vitamin D supplements and increasing the vitamin D levels impacted their symptoms. That said, this is yet another area that is interesting for more study about the impact of Vitamin D on health.

Alright Already, Where Do I Get Some?

Get some from three places: food, sunlight and supplements. Most foods do not contain vitamin D. Some fatty fish have it (like salmon) and fish liver oils are a good source (Yuck!). Beef liver, cheese and egg yolks also have some amount of vitamin D. Cereals and milk are often fortified with vitamin D. In fact, two glasses of vitamin D fortified milk a day gives enough vitamin D for people up to the age 50. Supplements are a bit harder to figure out. There is a lot of controversy about whether the body can really use supplements of vitamin D (especially without added calcium). The jury is still out on whether taking supplements is an effective way to counter vitamin D deficiency. Don't go all vitamin D crazy either. High levels of vitamin D are unhealthy. The sun is your best bet. Simply make sure you spend a little bit of time (around 15 minutes) outside each day. Just having your hands and face exposed during that time is enough. Don't overdo it though. Be careful of skin cancer, and be sure that you are not getting overexposed to the sun either.

How Do I Get Outside?

It may seem like a dumb question, but figuring out how to get outside is a challenge for many people. If you work in an office building and live in a neighborhood where you drive everywhere, finding time during the week to be outside is a real challenge. The most obvious way to do it is to go for a short walk at lunch. You get the health benefits of walking combined with the benefits of vitamin D. If you can't do that, you'll have to be creative. You can get your vitamin D exposure in parking lots (just park further away or walk around a bit). You can also just find a nice outdoor spot to make a few phone calls during the day. I like to make all those calls when you know you'll be on hold outside. Brainstorm a few ways to get yourself outside during your day.

The Problems with Vitamin D Deficiency Research

After reading all that, it seems like a great idea for everyone to focus on getting more vitamin D. Not so fast. It gets complicated. Here are some factors, pointed out in a National Institutes of Health (NIH) review of vitamin D, that make the "Should I take vitamin D supplements?" question difficult:

Many vitamins need to have other chemicals or vitamins present to be of any good. For example, taking vitamin D supplements without any added calcium may be a waste. Most studies haven't measured both calcium and vitamin D together.

Vitamin levels can vary widely in rats and probably do in people too. In other words, a person's vitamin D levels could shift over time and that shift hasn't been factored in studies either.

Complex factors could impact vitamin D deficiency including the time of year (less sunlight exposure in winter), the latitude (in higher latitudes, the sunlight is weaker and produces less vitamin D), physical activity levels, diet, etc.

The current tests for vitamin D levels have a lot of variation in them.

We don't have any real evidence that keeping vitamin D levels in the normal range actually prevents illness or disease.

We don't know what target vitamin D levels should be in people with various conditions.

People with illnesses probably go outside less. Lower vitamin D levels might be a result of a chronic illness, not a cause.

Illness (and medications) might interact with how the body produces vitamin D, causing a vitamin D deficiency.

Conclusion

If you get outside daily and have some exposure to sunlight, your vitamin D levels are probably okay. If you are inside a lot, it isn't a bad idea to focus on spending a few extra minutes outside each day. If you have an illness or just can't get out, consider asking your doctor to check your vitamin D levels. After all, 40% of men and 50% adults are thought to be vitamin D deficient. Of course, the solution is the same — just spend a little bit of time outside each day.

Chapter 8 - Do I Need Vitamins?

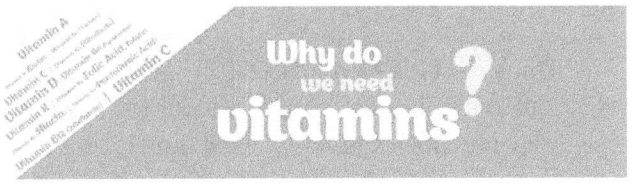

The questions about which vitamins a person should take is complicated, and I am not going to get into vitamin recommendations here. But what I am going to do is help you navigate the world of vitamin recommendations and supplements -- that way you'll be equipped with the right questions to ask your doctor or other health professional. Here are some basic questions and thoughts about vitamins and supplements to help you decide what vitamin recommendations you should follow:

Am I Taking Any Medications? Medications can change how your body processes nutrients, which can cause deficiencies in certain types of vitamins. Be sure to ask your doctor if you should take any vitamins along with your medications. You can also check Drug A-Z to find out yourself about the medications you are taking (then, remember to still check with you doctor as well).

What Do I Eat? If you eat a wide variety (5+ servings) of fruits and vegetables every day, chances are you are getting almost all the vitamins you need from your food (the best place to get vitamins). If you are not eating that well, you have a choice -- take vitamins to make up for the difference, or start eating healthier. My recommendation is to start eating healthier, because no matter how many vitamins you take, you'll still not be able to get the same quality of nutrients as you can from real food.

Do You Get Out Much? Vitamin D is becoming more and more important as researchers study this vitamin. If you are not outside at least for 15 minutes or so every day, or if you have concerns about skin cancer and always cover up - you may need some vitamin D supplementation. Your doctor can run a test to see your vitamin D levels and figure out what you may need.

Are You Pregnant? If you are pregnant, or planning to get pregnant, vitamins are a good idea. Here are some nutritional needs for pregnancy, but let your OB/GYN help guide you if you have any questions.

Of course, you're likely to hear about hundreds of wonderful things that vitamins and supplements can do and diseases they can prevent. Some of these claims might be true, and some clearly aren't. Use common sense, get advice and remember to eat real, healthy food to get your vitamins and minerals if possible. Also, keep in mind that taking too much of a vitamin or mineral can be harmful to you, so speak about the correct dosing with your doctor.

Beta Carotene and Cancer

Your body takes beta-carotene from foods and supplements and produces vitamin A. Wouldn't it be great if taking a beta-carotene supplement could help reduce your risk of cancer?

Given everything we known about antioxidants and vitamins, it seems likely that upping your daily intake of beta-carotene would be a good thing, cancer-risk wise. Here's what researchers found:

Researchers got 7,600 women over the age of 40 to take a beta-carotene supplement or a placebo every other day (the supplement was 50 milligrams of beta-carotene).

They then monitored the women in the study for 9 years. In that time, 624 of the women in the study developed some type of cancer (with 176 dying from cancer).

After looking at the data, researchers found no link between cancer risk and whether people were taking a placebo or the beta-carotene study. Bottom line: For the women in this study (over aged 40), beta-carotene had no effect on cancer risk.

In a separate study, researchers looked at the effects of beta-carotene on cancer risk in people who smoked. This study covered 29,133 male smokers who took 20 milligrams of beta-carotene, a placebo, a form of vitamin E or both beta-carotene and vitamin E.

For the men who took beta-carotene only, there was an 18% increase in their rate of lung cancer and an 8% increase in overall mortality.

In other words, for these men who smoked cigarettes, beta-carotene increased their risk for lung cancer and their overall risk of death over a 5- to 8-year period.

So it looks like beta-carotene is a bit of a bust for cancer prevention and can, in fact, be potentially dangerous in people who smoke. To avoid worrying about these types of issues, get your nutrients from real food, not from supplements.

Vitamin E for Longevity?

Can Vitamin E Help Prevent Cancer?

When I think of vitamins, I don't think about cancer prevention, I think about my mom putting a pin in a big capsule when I was a kid and squeezing the contents onto a bun. But vitamin E has a good reputation as a cancer fighter. What happens when research looks into the claim that vitamin E can prevent cancer?

If you took a vitamin E supplement every other day for 9 years, would your cancer risk change? That is the question that researchers wanted to answer with a group of 7,600 women aged 40 or older. The women were randomly divided into a group that took a vitamin E supplement (600 international units of alpha-tocopherol a.k.a. "vitamin E") or a placebo (other women in the study took vitamin C or beta-carotene). The result? The cancer risk for the vitamin E takers was the same as the placebo group. So, according to these data, vitamin E does not protect against cancer.

OK, but what about men? There is an ongoing study of 14,641 physicians. One of the things being tested was the impact of vitamin E on prostate cancer risk. One group of the physicians were given a vitamin E supplement every other day (400IU of vitamin E) and another group was given a placebo (another group took vitamin C). After 10 years, there was no difference in the risk for cancer and prostate cancer between the vitamin C takers and the placebo takers.

So, in both these studies, neither men nor women seemed to benefit from taking supplements of vitamin E, in terms of cancer risk. It could be that vitamin E has other benefits, but it seems, based on these data, that cancer prevention is not an apparent benefit of taking vitamin E supplements.

Vitamin C - A Myth?

Does Vitamin C Prevent Colds?

Vitamin C has long been held as the "cold prevention" vitamin. If we feel a little sick or if the cold season is coming on, we might start taking a vitamin C supplement for keep from getting sick. But does this really work? Where is the evidence about vitamin C and preventing colds?

The theory that vitamin C can help prevent colds comes from the idea that vitamin C gives the immune system "a boost." But does that boost really matter?

Researchers looked at studies of vitamin C where people took at least 200 milligrams of vitamin C daily in the form of a supplement and people were randomly placed in a placebo or vitamin C group. They then pooled the studies using a technique known as "meta-analysis." Here's what they found:

In 29 studies involving 11,077 people, the risk of developing cold symptoms during the study period was the same regardless of whether people were taking a daily supplement of vitamin C or a placebo. This was true for almost every group of people studied. There were a few exceptions:

People undergoing extreme physical exercise (marathon runners) or people exposed to extreme cold (skiers and soldiers in arctic weather) were half as likely to come down with cold symptoms if they were taking a vitamin C supplement.

Children taking a vitamin C supplement had shorter colds by 13% and adults taking a vitamin C supplement had shorter colds by 8%.

That said, overall there wasn't an effect of vitamin C on the number of colds or the severity of the cold (even using huge megadoses, like 4 grams) when someone starting coming down with a cold. Bottom line, vitamin C seems like a "bust" for preventing and managing colds.

I Have a Special Gift for My Readers

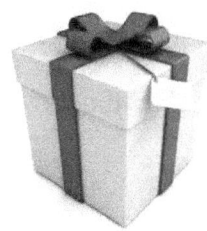

I appreciate my readers for without them I am just another author attempting to make a difference. If my book has made a favorable impression please leave me an honest review. Thank you in advance for you participation.

My readers and I have in common a passion for the written word as well as the desire to learn and grow from books.

My special offer to you is a massive ebook library that I have compiled over the years. It contains hundreds of fiction and non-fiction ebooks in Adobe Acrobat PDF format as well as the Greek classics and old literary classics too.

In fact, this library is so massive to completely download the entire library will require over 5 GBs open on your desktop.

Use the link below and scan all of the ebooks in the library. You can select the ebooks you want individually or download the entire library.

The link below does not expire after a given time period so you are free to return for more books rather than clog your desktop. And feel free to give the link to your friends who enjoy reading too.

I thank you for reading my book and hope if you are pleased that you will leave me an honest review so that I can improve my work and or write books that appeal to your interests.

Okay, here is the link…

http://tinyurl.com/special-readers-promo

PS: If you wish to reach me personally for any reason you may simply write to mailto:support@epubwealth.com.

I answer all of my emails so rest assured I will respond.

Meet the Author

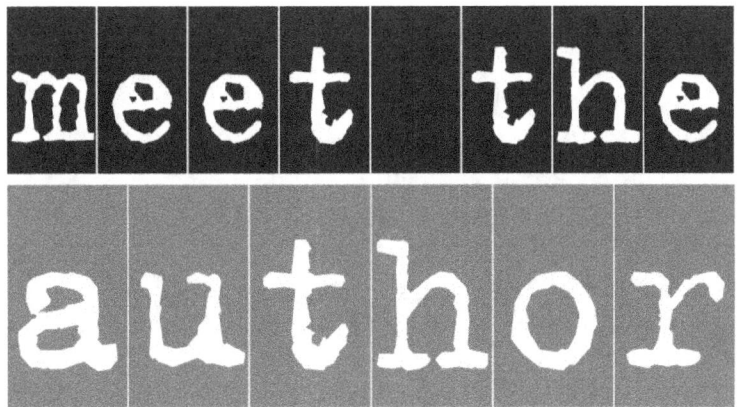

Dr. Noah Pranksky is a research behavioral scientist for Applied Mind Sciences. His research involves many aspects of the human mind including relationships, energy psychology, and various protocols and modalities relating to treatment and cure of various mental maladies.

He and his wife Marianne reside in Portland, Oregon.

Visit some of his websites

http://www.AddMeInNow.com
http://www.AppliedMindSciences.com
http://www.AppliedWebInfo.com
http://www.BookbuilderPLUS.com
http://www.BookJumping.com
http://www.EmailNations.com
http://www.EmbarrassingProblemsFix.com
http://www.ePubWealth.com
http://www.ForensicsNation.com
http://www.ForensicsNationStore.com
http://www.FreebiesNation.com
http://www.HealthFitnessWellnessNation.com
http://www.Neternatives.com
http://www.PrivacyNations.com
http://www.RetireWithoutMoney.org
http://www.SurvivalNations.com
http://www.TheBentonKitchen.com
http://www.Theolegions.org
http://www.VideoBookbuilder.com